Juicing and Smoothies for Health & Weight Loss

The Juicing and Smoothie Bible

Tammy Moore

This Page Intentionally Left Blank

Legal & Disclaimer

The information contained in this book is not designed to replace or take the place of any form of medicine or professional medical advice. The information in this book has been provided for educational and entertainment purposes only.

The information contained in this book has been compiled from sources deemed reliable, and it is accurate to the best of the Author's knowledge; however, the Author cannot guarantee its accuracy and validity and cannot be held liable for any errors or omissions. Changes are periodically made to this book. You must consult your doctor or get professional medical advice before using any of the suggested remedies, techniques, or information in this book.

Upon using the information contained in this book, you agree to hold harmless the Author from and against any damages, costs, and expenses, including any legal fees potentially resulting from the application of any of the information provided by this guide. This disclaimer applies to any damages or injury caused by the use and application, whether directly or indirectly, of any advice or information presented, whether for breach of contract, tort, negligence, personal injury, criminal intent, or under any other cause of action.

You agree to accept all risks of using the information presented inside this book. You need to consult a professional medical practitioner in order to ensure you are both able and healthy enough to participate in this program.

Table of Contents

Introduction

I decided to write this book as a result of catching mononucleosis (also known as glandular fever, mono, & the kissing disease). I wanted to pass along many of the lessons I have learned about health and how juicing has helped me in my life. I was incorrectly diagnosed with lymphoma cancer, but this misdiagnosis made me study how juicing can heal someone from the inside out. It was one of the best scares of my life, as now I juice at least once a day. I am also very fortunate that my "other job", when I am not authoring, has a fresh juice place nearby in which I am able to buy any mix of juice I like. The place I buy the juice from uses one of the same juicers that I have at home!! My readings revealed that juicing is a good way to help fix the digestive system and rebuild one's immune system. I decided I would buy a juicer and start juicing right away. Later I realized there are a few things to consider when buying a juicer which I will cover later in this book. At that time I was juicing 3-5 times per day. I started to get great energy and I could feel my body doing all it could to fight off the virus. Since that time I continue to juice 1-2 times a day, and vary which juice blends I use to keep myself healthy and strong. My body recovered a bit slowly due to my age, but faster than all the doctor's expectations. Since my full recovery I also noticed I rarely get sick. If I get a sniffle or feel a slight fever it rarely lasts more than a day, while many others around me pass around the flu or the common cold and it seems to not affect me.

While drinking fruit juices is nothing new, and for years many people have been consuming these beverages. The rise in popularity of these juices has become inevitable as studies and industry analysis have shown that there has been a dramatic increase in the sales of juices and smoothies. Modern tastes accompanied with healthy living concerns have resulted in new and delicious combinations of different flavors while using fresh ingredients. It may also be attributed to the fact that juices and smoothies are nutritious, quick and portable, and can be a replacement for milkshakes or unhealthy beverages such as soda.

This is why juices continue to take the market by storm. It is bound to dominate the category for healthy beverages replacements. Near my office and most places I frequent I see healthy fresh juice places popping up everywhere, making it easier for me to get my 2nd juice of the day in after my morning juice routine. The best part, is I always look at what juicer they are using behind the counter and compare it with what I have at home.

However it is good to beware of over the counter consumer products that seem to appear as healthful beverages. Many giant manufacturers are using dairy products, refined sugars, and other ingredients that we as consumers may not be unaware. There is a chance that only a small amount of healthy ingredients are included in these pre-packaged juices.

How can you make sure that the juice you are going to drink is healthy enough? Make one for yourself using the freshest fruits, vegetables, seeds, and nuts.

Do not worry as I will help you within this eBook to guide you on the step by step process to come up with your own favorite juice concoction. You will be given options on what to use as ingredients, whether they are a fruits, vegetables, natural sweeteners and add-ons, depending on your preference. Aside from that you will have a choice to an easier and tastier way to maximize your well-being, refresh your system and rebuild your health.

You will have many options and recipes that you can try. Flip the pages and before you know it, you are already hooked on making your own healthy and delicious juices. If you enjoy this book please take the time to leave me a review on Amazon, I welcome your feedback. Happy reading!

Chapter 1 – Juicing for a Better Life!

More people already know that including a good amount of fruits and vegetables in their diet is better for their health. Unfortunately, there are still a lot of people who have a hard time incorporating it into their everyday meal. What's the problem? Today's modern busy schedules is one of the reasons people feel they do not have enough time. Take for example a simple salad preparation. Instead of preparing their own salad they will simply buy ready-made meals. And yet another reason is many people do not like the taste of vegetables at all. However, this should not be a reason to eliminate or avoid eating your fruits and vegetables. This is where juicing will really help you.

A simple but properly made juice can do wonders for the body. Aside from the benefit of providing you with the daily dose of fruits and vegetables in your diet, you can enjoy many health benefits as listed below:

1) **Help in losing weight:** drinking fresh juices will help you satisfy your sweet cravings. Also, since fruits and vegetables are called "thermogenic", they contain few calories which help in weight loss and weight management.

2) **Faster nutrient absorption and helps in your digestion:** since juices are solid foods that are already broken down, it would be easier for you to digest them and promotes healthy digestive system. It will also help in absorbing nutrients immediately making its distribution faster throughout your

system. This is the main benefit you want to take advantage of if you have a cold, virus, or issues with your digestive tract.

3) **Provides you with a youthful, glowing skin:** juices helps in removing toxins from your body hence providing your skin with a healthy and radiant glow.

4) **Prevents diseases and boosts your immune system:** antioxidants and phytonutrients present in your juice helps in preventing various diseases and make your immune system stronger. This also helps in revitalizing your body.

5) **Increases energy:** when the body has enough nutrients that it needs, the levels of pH is well-balanced hence you will feel more energized. Since the nutrients are utilized by your body instantly, people who "juice" reported that they have experienced a "boost of energy" at the time of drinking and increased energy levels throughout the day.

6) **Allow you to consume a great deal of fruits and vegetables in a healthier manner:** juicing is a guarantee that you can incorporate a good amount of these foods in your diet with the added benefit of convenience, tastes great, and helps in weight loss.

7) **Adding more fruits and vegetables variety in your diet:** if you eat your fruits and vegetables with simple salad preparations, chances are, you might get tired of the same old tastes. With juicing you will be able to add a variety of different produce

with the added benefit of making your own customer flavored concoction.

8) **Helps in keeping you hydrated:** consuming juice throughout the day helps in keeping your body hydrated. Since fruits and vegetables contain water, they also add fluids to your body to help keep you refreshed and quenched the whole day.

9) **Children can also have their daily dose of essential nutrients:** let us admit, it is often hard to get children to eat fruits and vegetables. However, with juicing, you will be able to let them consume fruits and vegetables while really enjoying the taste. Since juices are delicious, children are easily encouraged to consume more thus providing them the nutrients they need for their growing bodies. Plus it is quite fun to use the juicer and the children can help you while also learn the healthy habits of juicing.

10) **Boost your brain function:** There are many fruits and vegetables that help in giving your brain proper nutrients it needs to improve memory, improves brain power, and increases focus. It will always keep you active and alert.

11) **A perfect detoxifier:** Many people nowadays are always exposed to many chemicals, free-radicals and pollution which are all harmful to health. Consuming juices every day will help in detoxifying your body from these harmful items. Fruits and vegetables contain a great amount of detoxifying ingredients hence reducing the impact of these free radicals in your body.

These are just some of the great benefits juicing can provide your body. The following chapters will provide you information on how to create your own, perfectly delicious juices and other useful tips that should help make you love juicing even more!

Chapter 2 – Everything You Need To Know About Juicing

We have already covered the benefits juicing can bring to your body. This chapter will prepare you with the right tools, tips, and tricks to help you start juicing right away.

Getting Started

Yes, juicing is really easy but it does take some preparation time. You have to be a little patient and have some dedication to juicing, but believe me the benefits are worth it and the tastes are truly exceptional. Here are some of the key steps to get you started:

1) Selecting the type of juicer that is right for you.
2) Shop for the fresh ingredients that you will use. Make sure that you already have a grocery list and plan ahead so that you will know what type of fruits and vegetables you will be using.
3) In order to save time, prepare your fruits and vegetables the night before. You can wash, chop and store them in the fridge so that you will simply juice them on the next day. You might also want to assemble your equipment to further save time.
4) With everything ready you can easily juice in the morning. If you buy a slow juicer, you can juice the night before and put the juice in a container with a lid and drink in the morning.

Choosing the Essential Equipment

Most of the equipment needed to make smoothies and juices are almost all there in a well-equipped kitchen. There is no special equipment required but of course, it will all depend on what type of juicer or juicers you want to have in your kitchen.

There are basically 2 types of juicers or juice extractors available in the market. There is the masticating juicers and the centrifugal juicers.

Centrifugal juicer is where you will feed the produce through the spinning blade. It is fast, light weight and great with almost all fruits and vegetables. You don't even need to chop or slice the most produce because you will simply feed them in the tube. However, they are not too good when it comes to juicing leafy vegetables and can be a bit noisy. I have one of these, which I use to make juice fast, but I drink the juice right away.

Masticating juicers on the other hand, works by chewing or squeeze the produce with the use of a twin-gear. They are great with leafy vegetables, have a quiet operation, produce more pulp and can also be used for other purpose such as ice cream, nuts, and milk. However, they can slightly be more expensive, it is slower (thus the nick-name slow juicer) and produce usually has to be cut to smaller pieces before you can use it in order to prevent clogging. I have one of these that I use more often and use for most of my green vegetable juice mixes.

Remember that a juicer is different from a blender. The two pieces of equipment are often confused with one another. Take note that a juicer separates the pulp and the juice while a blender includes everything and nothing is removed or separated.

Aside from the juicers you also need other materials which I believe most people already have such as chopping board, knife, citrus press, apple corer, knives, strainer, and vegetable peelers. These are all secondary tools and not all need to be used for all juice preparation. Your juicer is the most important equipment in order to produce a healthy glass of juice, so decide slowly and wisely, but pick one and go get it quickly!!

How to make your own healthy juice:

1) Make sure that you wash your produce thoroughly. Unwashed fruits and vegetables might be contaminated with bacteria so it is important to keep them clean. It is also a good idea to find a really good fruit and vegetable cleaner. After rinsing my produce, I put them in a bucket of water and put a few drops of the cleaner into the water and let it soak for a few hours. Then dry off and put in the refrigerator.

2) If your juicer has a pulp basket, you may want to place a plastic bag so that you can easily clean it up once you are done.

3) Cut or chop your produce according to your juicer's instructions. There are some that require small

pieces while others don't require chopping at all. For optimum benefit, cut your fruits and vegetables when you are ready to make the juice. However, you can still prepare them before hand as long as they are stored properly.

4) Feed the produce through your juicer: if your juicer comes in one or more speed, make sure that you will decrease its speed especially when using softer fruits. Most of the juicers come with manuals to guide you on how to use the correct speed.

5) Re-juicing the pulp: check the pulp of your fruits or vegetables after you have juiced them once. If it is still damp, then you can place it back in your juicer and get more juice. Don't throw away the left-overs just yet!

6) Drink up! Now you already have your own juice. Consume as soon as possible. Take note that once you have already juiced your fruits and vegetables, they start losing their nutritional content. Juices that are stored properly can last for only until 2 days. So once you are done juicing, pour it in a glass, and enjoy! Don't forget to rinse and clean up your juicer once you are done.

7) The left over pulp can be used as a mulch in your garden now or plants now. I used it throughout my garden.

Chapter 3 – Common Ingredients for Making Juices and Smoothies

Juices and smoothies have become very trendy beverages nowadays. It is easy to make, all you need are your fruits or vegetables, for smoothies a base which can be water, yogurt, or milk, and blender or juicers. Since fruits and/or vegetables are the main ingredients in making these beverages, it helps in keeping yourself healthy and fit.

But before making your own beverage, here are the recommended fruits or vegetables that you can use and the benefits you can get from each of them:

Fruits

If you prefer fruits in your smoothies, you can use any fruit you want. But, you might want to consider the benefits of each individual fruit in your health. Take a look at the benefits of the following fruits commonly used in smoothies:

- **Berries-** Excellent source of antioxidants and phytochemicals. Rich in fiber, Vitamins A and C, magnesium and potassium.
  - o **Blueberry- is** ranked as one of the fruits with highest antioxidant capacities. A study shows that blueberries can improve memory. It contains Vitamin C, iron, phosphorus, calcium, manganese, magnesium, vitamin K, and zinc. Blueberry is very helpful in maintaining healthy bones, managing

diabetes, preventing cancer and heart diseases.

o **Strawberry-** like other berries, contains Vitamin C, which boosts the immune system. It can also reduce inflammation of the joints which may cause arthritis.

o **Blackberry-** a delicious and versatile fruit which contains vitamins A, B1, B2, B3, B6, C, E, and K. It also contains calcium, iron, magnesium, phosphorous, potassium, zinc, amino acids and antioxidants. Blackberry reduces the risk of having stroke and atherosclerosis, aids in constipation and digestion problems, prevents the development of lung and colon cancer. It is also useful in maintaining healthy eyesight, bones, and skin.

o **Raspberry-** contains rich amounts of antioxidants, phytonutrients, fiber, magnesium, iron, potassium, zinc, and vitamins C, E, and K. Raspberry improves the immune system, slows down aging, prevents the development of cancer, controls inflammation, maintains healthy eyesight, improves blood circulation and cardiovascular health.

o **Kiwi-** is also called Chinese gooseberry, kiwi berries or kiwi for short, is a nutritional powerhouse. It is rich in folic acid, high in fiber, and an extraordinary source of chromium.

- **Citrus Fruits-** refreshing, nutritious, and high in Vitamin C. The Vitamin C found in these fruits strongly improves iron absorption from food. They also have flavonoids and antioxidants that protect against heart disease and neutralize free radicals.
  - o **Pineapple-** low in calories, low in sodium, fat-free, and cholesterol-free. Pineapples boost the immune system, bone strength, digestion, and eye health. It reduces blood clotting and also reduces the mucus in the throat and nose, thus, preventing common colds and sinus inflammation.
  - o **Orange-** has no fat, cholesterol, or sodium. Orange helps prevent cancer and kidney diseases, lowers cholesterol, and boosts heart and eye health. It also relieves constipation and regulates high blood pressure.
  - o **Lemon-** very low in calories, a rich source of calcium, potassium, Vitamin C, and pectin fiber. Lemon helps to cure fever, indigestion and constipation. It can be used to improve skin, hair, dental health, and often used in the treatment of arthritis, cholera, and malaria.
  - o **Grapefruit-** contains good sugar, phosphorus, vitamin C, potassium, and lycopene. Grapefruits are low in calories and rich in fiber. It also contains bioflavonoids

14

that protects against cancer and heart diseases.

o **Passion Fruit** – they are great sources of vitamin A and C and have sweet and sour taste. They are also rich sources of antioxidants minerals and fibers which helps in proper digestion and protects the colon.

- **Fleshy Fruit**- rich in fiber, vitamin C, and potassium. Since they are rich in potassium, they are good in maintaining normal blood pressure and they have a protective effect against hypertension.

  o **Banana**- rich in potassium and pectin. It contains vitamins A, B6, C, manganese, magnesium, folate, iron, and protein. It helps in maintaining normal blood pressure, prevention of asthma, heart diseases, and cancer development. It is also used in the treatment of diabetes and diarrhea. Bananas also contain tryptophan, which preserves memory and boosts mood. Just remember that if you will be using this ingredient use a blender to thicken up your juice. Don't use this in your juicer.

  o **Apple**- extremely rich in flavonoids, antioxidants, and dietary fibers. Many different research shows that apples can improve neurological health, reduce the risk of stroke and diabetes, prevent dementia and breast cancer, and lower bad cholesterol.

- o **Cucumber-** excellent source of vitamin K and molybdenum. It contains copper, potassium, manganese, and vitamins B and C which prevent nutrient deficiencies. Cucumber has anti-inflammatory as well as antioxidant properties. It also reduces risk against cancer, helps freshen breath, and plays a role in brain and heart health.
- o **Watermelon-** made up mostly of water. But it also contains significant levels of vitamins A, B6, C, antioxidants, amino acids, and lycopene. It is also low in sodium and calories. It reduces the risk of developing asthma and cancer. It aids in digestion, reduces inflammation, helps in maintaining skin moisture, and prevents dehydration.
- o **Cantaloupe-** contains high levels of vitamins A, B6, C, potassium, niacin, fiber, and folic acid. Cantaloupe reduces the risk of cancer, kidney diseases and gastrointestinal problems, relieves anxiety and stress, and boosts the immune system. It also reduces inflammation, prevents arthritis, and protects skin against harmful toxins.
- o **Pear-** rich in fiber, antioxidants, flavonoids, vitamins B2, C, E, copper and potassium. Pear prevents the growth and development of cancer, lowers blood cholesterol, reduce the risk of stroke, and controls diabetes.

- **Stone Fruit-** rich in vitamins A, C, and K. Stone fruits help strengthen bones, relieve constipation, sharpen eyesight, and form collagen.
  - **Peach-** is rich in vitamins A, C, E, K, and B complex. It also contains fibers, bioactive compounds and potassium. Beta carotene in peach protects and improves eyesight. It improves skin and cardiovascular health, maintains normal blood pressure, controls high cholesterol, aids in digestion, protects against anemia, reduces inflammation and prevents cancer.
  - **Nectarine-** is closely related to peaches, nectarines contain antioxidants, vitamins A and C, potassium, beta carotene, lutein, bioflavonoids and fibers. It has no saturated fats and is low in calories. Nectarine aids in digestion, helps in maintaining normal blood pressure, reduces risk against cancer, and improves heart health.
  - **Apricot-** contains vitamins A, C, K, E, niacin, potassium, copper, manganese, magnesium, phosphorous, and fiber. Apricot aids in treating anemia, asthma and cancer, helps prevent osteoporosis, aids in digestion and bowel movement, reduces the risk of heart diseases, boosts metabolism, cures fever, and essential for the growth and development of bones.
  - **Plum-** is an excellent source of vitamins A, B1, B2, B3, B6, C, E, and K. Plums also

contains folate, potassium, fluoride, phosphorous, magnesium, iron, calcium, and zinc. It is also rich in fiber and contains very low calories. Plums are great in relieving constipation and digestive problems. It reduces the risk of having a stroke and cancer, prevents diabetes, maintains normal blood pressure, and improves brain memory.

o **Mango-** is a rich in prebiotic dietary fiber, flavonoid, pectin, vitamins A, B6, C, E, and potassium. Mango lowers cholesterol, promotes eye and skin health, improves digestion, prevents stroke and cancer, and controls diabetes.

o **Avocado-** is a rich source of pantothenic acid and fiber. It also contains vitamins B6, C, E, K, potassium, copper, and folate. Avocado helps reduce blood cholesterol level, decrease the risk of heart diseases, regulates blood sugar and blood pressure, improves vision, digestion and the immune system, and prevents cancer. Just like the banana, use a blender to thicken up your juice. Don't use this in your juicer.

Vegetables

If you want to use vegetables in your smoothie and juices, you need to know what benefits you can get from vegetables as well. Like fruits, vegetables are very healthy, which is why it is very suitable for those who want a very refreshing, yet very nutritious drink. Take a look at the following vegetables and learn about their benefits:

- **Yellow/Orange Vegetables-** contains zeaxanthin, flavonoids, potassium, vitamin A and C, and lycopene. These vegetables fight harmful free radicals in the body, boosts the immune system, promotes collagen formation, and lowers blood pressure and cholesterol.
  - o **Carrots-** rich in vitamins A, B8, C, K, pantothenic acid, potassium, iron, copper, folate, and manganese. Carrots improve vision, promotes healthier skin, prevents infections, stroke, heart diseases and cancer, and cleanses the body.
  - o **Squash-** rich in beta carotene and lutein. Squash also contains vitamin C; iron; foliate; low in carbohydrates, fat, and calories; and is cholesterol free.
  - o **Tomato-** excellent source of vitamins A, B6, C, E, and K. It also contains biotin, copper, potassium, molybdenum, manganese, fiber, niacin, phosphorus, and folate. Tomatoes promote eye, skin, and hair health, help to prevent cancer and kidney diseases, regulate blood pressure, maintain strong bones, and repair damage caused by smoking.

- **Green Vegetables-** an excellent source of fiber, carotenoids, and folate. These vegetables also contain vitamins C, K, iron, and calcium, and act as antioxidants.

o **Kale**- rich in protein, fiber, vitamins A, C, K, folate, lutein, phosphorus, potassium, calcium, zinc, and zeaxanthin. Kale helps control diabetes, decrease the risk of cardiovascular diseases, regulate blood pressure, prevent cancer, improve bone health and digestion, and promote skin and hair health.

o **Parsnip**- contains high levels of magnesium, phosphorous, potassium, zinc, iron, fiber, protein, and vitamins B, C, E, and K. Parsnip reduces the risk of developing diabetes and heart diseases, regulates blood pressure and cholesterol levels, and improves digestion and metabolism.

o **Spinach**- an excellent source of vitamins A, B1, B2, B6, C, K, iron, folate, copper, phosphorus, fiber, magnesium, zinc, protein, calcium, potassium, and choline. Spinach helps control diabetes, prevents asthma and cancer, regulates blood pressure, promotes skin and hair health, and maintains strong bone health.

o **Parsley**- rich in vitamins A, B6, B12, C, K, thiamin, riboflavin, niacin, pantothenic acid, choline, calcium, iron, magnesium, manganese, phosphorous, zinc, copper, potassium, and foliates. Parsley helps to control diabetes and rheumatoid arthritis, prevents inflammation, osteoporosis and cancer, and strengthens the immune system.

o **Broccoli**- a good source of fiber, pantothenic acid, vitamins A, B1, B6, E, phosphorus, copper, potassium, choline, protein, iron, zinc, calcium, niacin, and selenium. Broccoli helps in reducing allergic reactions, improve bone and heart health, prevents constipation, improves digestion, maintains blood sugar levels, reduces cholesterol, and is a powerful antioxidant.

o **Cabbage**- an excellent source of vitamins B1, B6, C, K, manganese, fiber, copper, calcium, potassium, folate and antioxidants. Cabbage improves eyes and heart health, the immune system, and the digestive system. It is also known to prevent cancer and inflammation, improve mental function, maintain blood pressure, and build strong bone health.

o **Lettuce**- is rich in vitamins A, B1, B2, B6, C, E, & K, copper, iron, calcium, phosphorous, chromium, potassium, biotin, magnesium, antioxidants and pantothenic acid. Lettuce lowers cholesterol levels, aids in insomnia, improves brain health, and prevents inflammation.

o **Celery**-is a good source of vitamins A, V2, B6, C, and K, pantothenic acid, potassium, folate, fibers, manganese, phosphorus, calcium and magnesium. Celery reduces inflammation, regulates alkaline balance in the body, aids in digestion, reduces bad cholesterol, regulates blood pressure, prevents cancer, and promotes eye health.

o **Cilantro**- an excellent source of thiamin and zinc. It also contains vitamins A, B6, C, E, K, calcium, iron, magnesium, fiber, riboflavin, niacin, folate, pantothenic acid, copper, potassium, and manganese. Cilantro also has antioxidant, anti-inflammatory, anti-fungal, anti-bacterial, and anti-diabetic properties. It also helps in reducing risk of cardiovascular diseases, improves digestion, lowers blood sugar level, and improves sleep quality.

o **Chard**- is rich in vitamins A, B2, B6, C, E, and K, copper, magnesium, manganese, iron, fiber, choline, calcium, phosphorus, protein, and potassium. Chard prevents cancer, controls diabetes, lowers blood pressure, and prevents osteoporosis.

The above fruits and vegetables are the more common, but only some of the produce that you can use in making your own juices. You can use them individually or more commonly make a mix of several fruits and vegetables. It will just depend on your taste, preference, and specific health needs.

Chapter 4 – Juicing and Smoothie Facts

Before you start making your own juice and smoothies, here are some frequently asked questions regarding juicing and smoothie-making that you may want to consider as you adapt them into your lifestyle:

1. How much fruit and vegetables do I need to consume each day?

    -   Because the presence of instant and processed foods have been increasing overtime, consuming fruits and vegetables are therefore essential to be added to our daily routines. The average intake requirement for adults should be at least 7 servings (5 servings of vegetables and 2-4 servings of fruits). Juices and smoothies would allow you to boost your fruit and vegetable intake every day because it's easy to make and consume, which will in turn, help you to meet your daily nutritional needs. Remember that a glass (8 oz.) of vegetable juice contains 3-4 servings of vegetables while a glass (8 oz.) of vegetable smoothie contains 2-3 servings of vegetables.

2. What is the difference between juicing and blending (smoothies)? Is there a better choice?

- Both juices and smoothies provide the health benefits we need. Juicing is a process where insoluble fiber coming from fruits and veggies is discarded and all that would be extracted is the water and the nutrients from the produce. This means that the juice would be more potent and would be introduced and absorbed directly into our blood streams that would help you get the nutrients faster. On the other hand, smoothies would contain all the produce, fiber, skin and all, which would help make you feel fuller for a longer time and could assist you in avoiding excessive eating. If you are looking to detox, juicing would be better because they are rich in nutrients and restores the body at a cellular level. Smoothies are better if you're on a diet since it regulates your food consumption and would help you avoid unhealthy food intake and makes you feel full as mentioned before.

3. How do I start juicing and smoothie-making a lifestyle?

- First thing you need to invest in is a good juicer & a blender. There are a number of great juicers and blenders on the market that you can choose from. When juicing, remember to get the low speed juicers which would get the most out of your produce since it masticates and presses the juice, allowing you to get all the nutrients from it. Whereas high speed juicers would only break down some of the nutrients due to the excessive heat that comes with the high speed. For blending, you need to choose a powerful motor that can blend everything, including leafy vegetables without any trouble. Of course, it is best to get a blender and a juicer that could perform with minimal noise and high quality so they last a long time. They are important investments and you do not want to be paying twice.

- Second, make sure that you are buying fresh produce. It is best to get organic fruits and veggies if possible. If not, you can get any fresh clean looking produce in your local groceries, but make sure to soak them well. Rinse them in cold water and juice or blend before they spoil which for most is just a few days.

- Third, check the blender or juicer manufacturer's instructions before you use it. Every juicing and blending machine is different. So want to read up on the features and care of the devices and take care of your equipment well.

- Fourth, there's an abundance of juice and smoothie strategies available that you can choose from. Just remember to start something that's realistic and would complement your everyday activities. More importantly you have to give it time, you will see the results soon.

- Fifth, there is a rule of thumb when juicing or blending: Add the most delicate ingredients first like leafy vegetables and herbs, followed by soft vegetables and fruits, and finally finish with hard vegetables and fruits.

26

- Finally, consume the juice or smoothie within the day as it oxidizes the more it's exposed to air plus the nutrients are gradually decreasing. I often juice a bit for 2-days quantity and store in the refrigerator due to my schedule, but I make sure I finish within 2-days' time. You might want to consume once you are done preparing the juice.

4. Can juices and smoothies replace my meals?

- Like almost anything in life, juice and smoothie consumption should also be consumed in moderation. Having a balanced meal is crucial in getting the most out of juicing and blending. First, a smoothie should have ample amount of calories for it to be considered a meal. Second, going through a day with only juice in your stomach wouldn't be enough to get the energy you need to last the whole day. You still need to eat solid meals as well. A balanced diet of juice or smoothie, protein, whole grains and healthy fats would be best to get the most benefits for your health.

5. When is the right time to juice?

- If we are talking about the time of the day, the best time to drink your juice is when you don't have any food intake yet, about 30 minutes before you eat. This is because your stomach is hungry and it will absorb anything you eat or drink. Hence if you eat or drink foods that are unhealthy, your body will surely absorb those unhealthy elements. However, if you consume healthy foods, then of course, healthy elements will be absorbed in the body. Generally, drinking juices when your start your day will provide important carbs and nutrients that will fuel your body with energy for the day. On the latter part of the day, green juices are the best.

• Now, if you we talking about "the best time to start" juicing – it will all depend on you. Before embarking on a juicing diet, remember that you have to know the status of your health first. There are certain illnesses where juicing is not recommended. Ask your doctor first if you have any uncertainties so that you can be guided accordingly.

It's so easy to get into the habit of juicing and blending. Juices and smoothies could have a life-changing effect on your health and lifestyle. It's never too late to start living healthy and there's no better time to start than today.

Chapter 5 – Easy and Delicious Juicing and Smoothie Recipes

This chapter will reveal delicious and nutritious recipes for you to try out. As mentioned in the previous chapter, juicing helps in losing weight, detoxification, and provides good looking skin that will make you feel young and refreshed.

Go ahead and bring out your juicers or blenders and let's get juicing and blending!

Coconut Lime Detox Drink

Ingredients
- 2 handfuls of baby spinach
- 1/3 cup of freshly squeezed lime juice
- 3-4 tablespoons of freshly squeezed lemon juice
- 1 cup of coconut water
- 2 handfuls of ice (you can add more if you want)
- Maple syrup for tasting

Directions

Place all ingredients into your blender and blend until smooth. Add more water or ice to obtain desired consistency.

Grapefruit and Ginger Juice

Ingredients

- 1 orange

29

- 2 carrots
- 1/2 inch of ginger
- 1 ruby grapefruit

Directions

Wash produce well, peel your grapefruit and orange. Add ingredients to your juicer, serve and enjoy.

Berry and Chia Smoothie

Ingredients

- ½ cup of pomegranate juice (unsweetened)
- 1 cup of mixed berries (frozen)
- ½ tablespoon of chia seeds
- ½ cup of water

Directions

Combine all of the ingredients in your blender. Blend until it becomes smooth, serve and enjoy.

Vitamin C Smoothie

Ingredients

- ½ of cantaloupe
- 1 cup of strawberries
- 1 tomato
- 2 oranges
- Ice cube

Directions

Juice the oranges and combine it with the other ingredients in the blender. Blend with ice, serve and enjoy!

Cucumber and tomato juice

Ingredients

- 2 cups of diced cucumber
- A stalk of celery
- 3 ½ cups of tomatoes (chopped)
- ½ teaspoon of black pepper (ground)
- 3-4 drops of stevia (if desired)
- ¼ teaspoon of cayenne pepper
- ½ teaspoon of sea salt

Directions

Take your juicer if you prefer juice or blender if you prefer more of a smoothie with fiber and then put all of the cut veggies inside. Process until juiced or well blended. Add cayenne pepper, sea salt and black pepper. If you prefer your beverage to be a bit sweet, add stevia. Pour over glass and serve.

Beets and Celery Juice

Ingredients

- A small sized beet (diced)
- A bunch of cilantro

- A teaspoon of sea salt
- 4-5 celery stalks
- A cup of spinach (chopped coarsely)

Directions

Place all of the ingredients in your juicer. You can also blend them all together. Pour it in your glass and add a bit of lemon juice to taste.

Beets, Carrots, Cabbage, & Spinach with Pineapple, Orange, & Lemon

Ingredients

- 1 beet root
- 3 medium sized carrots
- 2 leaves of red cabbage
- 1/2 fruit of lemon
- 1 orange
- 2 handfuls of spinach
- ¼ of pineapple

Directions

Juice all of the ingredients in your juicer. Transfer to glass, stir and serve.

Healthy Cocktail

Ingredients

- 2 medium sized apples
- 1 cucumber
- 2 stalks of medium-sized celery
- 5 leaves of kale
- 1/2 a fruit of lemon
- 2 orange

Directions

Juice all of the ingredients in your juicer. Transfer to glass, stir and enjoy!

Watermelon and lemon Juice

Ingredients

- A cup of watermelon
- A teaspoon of mint leaves
- 1 lemon

Directions

Use your blender and place all ingredients. Blend well until you see a red mass inside. Add some crushed ice in your glass and pour the juice.

Green Power Juice

Ingredients

- A cup of sliced kale (around 3 leaves)

- 1 cucumber (sliced thick)
- 1 Granny Smith apple (cored then cut to chunks)
- 1/2 a cup of water
- A cup of green grapes (seedless)

Directions

Using your blender, add all of the ingredients then blend until it becomes smooth. Strain the juice and add water to thin if desired. Transfer to glass. Serve and enjoy!

Hydrating Juice

Ingredients

- 2 apples (preferably organic)
- 2-3 large cucumbers (preferably organic)
- ¼ of beet or you can also use a handful of fresh strawberries
- Mint for garnish

Directions

Juice all of the ingredients using your juicer. Transfer to glass and add ice. Garnish with mint. Serve and

Colorful Veggie Juice

Ingredients

- 4 sliced tomatoes

- 3 medium-sized carrots
- 1 to 2 sliced and seeded red bell peppers
- A bunch of celery
- 2 heads of lettuce (Romaine)
- A handful of fresh parsley and cilantro
- A cucumber (chopped and peeled)
- An inch of ginger root
- 2 lemons (peeled)

Directions

Juice all of the veggies in your juicer.

Root Veggie Juice

Ingredients

- 1 beet root
- 1 sweet potato
- 10 medium-sized carrots

Directions

Juice all of the root veggies in your juicer. First the beet then sweet potato and carrots. Stir and place them on a glass. Add ice and a bit of sweetener if you want.

Red Detox Juice (My Personal Favorite)

Ingredients

- 1 medium sized beet (peeled and quartered)
- 4 medium-sized carrots (sliced and cleaned well)
- 1-2 medium sized apple (quartered)
- 1 tablespoon of fresh ginger (chopped and peeled)

Directions

Using your Juicer (the reason I quarter the ingredients is to make it easier to get into smaller juicers) place in all of the ingredients and juice completely. Transfer to glass and serve. You can refrigerate the remaining juice for up to 2 days. I do this 2-3 times a week as my regular morning juice.

Pomegranate and Citrus Juice

Ingredients

- 3 oranges
- 3 medium carrots
- 1 large pink grapefruit
- 1 pomegranate
- 1/2 of a lime

Directions

Juice all of the ingredients in your juicer. Stir and place them in a glass or mason jar. Add ice if you like chilled. Best if consumed immediately.

Healthy Red Mary

Ingredients

- 4 stalks of celery
- 1 jalapeno (seeded) – if you like spicy
- 1 tomato – if you do not like spicy
- ¼ of lemon (peeled)
- 1/2 of a cucumber
- ¼ cup of cilantro
- 2 large cilantro

Directions

Juice all of the ingredients in your juicer.

Cucumber and Spinach Juice

Ingredients

- 1 cucumber
- 2 handfuls of spinach
- 1 apple
- 4 medium-sized carrots
- 1/2 of a lemon

Directions

Juice all of the ingredients in your juicer. Best if consumed immediately.

Chard and Kale Juice

Ingredients

- 2 to 3 leaves of Swiss Chard
- 3 carrots
- 1 cucumber
- 1/2 of a lemon
- 2 Granny Smith apples
- A bunch of kale
- A bunch of baby spinach

Directions

Juice all of the veggies in your juicer.

Spicy and Healthy Green Juice

Ingredients

- ¼ cup of fresh parsley
- 1 stalk of celery (cut to chunks)
- 1 small cucumber (peeled)
- Juice of 1 lemon
- 2 large handfuls of baby spinach
- An inch of ginger (peeled)
- Ice cubes and water

Directions

Using your blender, place all of the ingredients until it becomes frothy and smooth. Transfer to glass and serve immediately. Consume right away before the juice starts to separate.

Energy Juice

Ingredients

- 1 pear
- An inch of peeled ginger
- 1 green apple
- 1/2 a lemon
- 3 carrots

Directions

Juice all of the ingredients in your juicer.

Pizza Juice

Ingredients

- 1 yellow and 1 orange bell pepper
- 1/3 of yellow onion
- 4-5 roma tomatoes
- 10-15 leaves of basil
- 1 peeled garlic clove
- A bunch of kale

- A handful of raw cashew nuts

Directions

Juice all of the ingredients in your juicer except the cashew. Stir then place them in the blender together with the cashew. Blend well until smooth.

Basic Ginger and Mango Lemonade

Ingredients

- 1 lemon
- A thin slice of ginger
- Zest of a lemon
- ½ of a mango
- A tablespoon of agave nectar
- Ice cubes

Directions

Using your blender, place all the ingredients and blend well. Add a piece or two of lemon to garnish and serve.

Citrus Zinger

Ingredients

- Peeled 1/2 of a red grapefruit
- 3 orange (peeled)
- 1 apple

Directions

Juice all of the ingredients in your juicer.

Avocado with Lemon Lime Smoothie

Ingredients:

- ½ an avocado
- 1 lemon (peeled)
- 1 cup of water or coconut water
- ½ tablespoon of honey (optional)
- ½ cup of ice cubes (optional)

Directions:

Combine all of the ingredients in your blender. Blend until it becomes smooth and serve.

Collard Greens with Lime and Mango

Ingredients:

- 2 tablespoons of fresh lime juice
- 2 cups of collard greens (stemmed and chopped)
- 1 ½ cup of mango (frozen)
- 1 cup of green grapes

Directions:

Place all the ingredients in your blender. Blend until smooth and serve.

Chapter 6 – 7 or 14 Day Juicing Challenge

Now that you already know the great benefits of juicing plus the knowledge on how to prepare them, it's about time that you try and take the 14-day juicing challenge. Juicing can also be a good way to lose weight because it stops your cravings for foods that are rich in calories and juices provide most of your vitamins and minerals needs. Just a word of advice: remember to check with your health physician first before embarking on any diet. Check the status of your health and ask your physician if it's safe for you to try out the juicing diet because not all individuals are in the right health to start the juicing diet. It is also important to remember that not all diets have the same result with every individual. So if you think that you are not losing weight fast enough, give it some time. Just be patient and think about why it is not yet working for you.

Here's a simple 7-day plan that you can follow for up to 14-days (two week). You can refer back to the recipes in the previous chapters.

Day 1:

- Upon waking up drink hot water with lime, mint, or lemon
- Start your day with the Green Power Juice as your breakfast.

42

- For lunch and dinner, choose from the Green Juice recipes like Chard and Kale Juice or Cucumber and Spinach Juice.
- End the day with mint tea

Day 2:

- Upon waking up drink hot water with lime, mint, or lemon
- Start your day with the Berry and Chia Smoothie as your breakfast.
- For lunch and dinner, choose from the Beets recipes like Beets and Celery Juice or Beets, Carrots and Cabbage Juice.
- End the day with mint tea

Day 3:

- Upon waking up drink hot water with lime, mint or lemon
- Start your day with the Energy Juice as your breakfast.
- For lunch and dinner, choose from Avocado with Lime or Collard Greens
- End the day with mint tea

Day 4:

- Upon waking up drink hot water with lime, mint, or lemon

- Start your day with the Hydrating Juice as your breakfast.
- For lunch and dinner, choose from the Coconut Lime Detox or Vitamin C Smoothie.
- End the day with mint tea

Day 5:

- Upon waking up drink hot water with lime, mint, or lemon
- Start your day with the Red Detox as your breakfast.
- For lunch and dinner, choose from Pizza Juice or the Spicy and Healthy Green Juice.
- End the day with mint tea

Day 6:

- Upon waking up drink hot water with lime, mint, or lemon
- Start your day with the Root Veggie Juice as your breakfast.
- For lunch and dinner, choose from Colorful Veggie or Healthy Red Mary.
- End the day with mint tea

Day 7:

- Upon waking up drink hot water with lime, mint, or lemon
- Start your day with the Cucumber and Tomato as your breakfast.

- For lunch and dinner, choose from the Basic Ginger Juice or Citrus Zinger
- End the day with mint tea

NOTE: These are just suggested juices that you can combine in a day. I recommend you have a mix of fruit juices and mostly veggie juices for each day to get the proper mix of vitamins and minerals. You can modify the menu to your taste throughout the duration of your juicing diet.

Repeat the 7-Day plan about for 14-days if you want to lose more weight or it takes most of the first 7-days to start to see results. Then start to mix a healthy regular diet (Take a look at my "Rebuild Your Health with a Mediterranean Diet" book if you are looking for a tasty way to eat healthy) with a morning and either an afternoon or after dinner juice or smoothie. This will help you maintain your weight and continue to rebuild your health.

Tips that you should remember:

- If there are ingredients that do not appeal to your taste, you can always substitute them with a different ingredient. For example, if you are not a fan of Kale, then go ahead and substitute them with spinach or broccoli. Be creative, adventurous, and just stay with it!
- As much as possible, in order to make this plan work, try not to eat solid foods for the whole 7 or 14 days. You might feel some strong cravings or maybe headaches, that's normal. Just stick with the plan. Prepare an extra juice if you are hungry or

drink tea. After 3 to 4 days, you will be feeling more energized and the headaches will disappear. This means that your body has started adapting to the change and this is a good indication. Keep up the good work and be remain patient.

- Remember to drink water after every juice drink. Try to consume at least 12-16 ounces of water after each juice to stay hydrated.
- Don't forget to prepare your hot to warm water with lemon, mint, or lime in order to cleanse your whole digestive system. This will help in giving you a great amount of energy that will last the whole day.
- It is recommended that you consume 4 to 6 juices a day that consists of 16-20 ounces per serving. You can choose from the recipes in this book. Once you get the hang of juicing, you can definitely create your own unique concoctions.
- In preparing your juices, always remember to wash and clean your produce thoroughly before juicing it. Clean your juicer after every use, this will prevent it from getting moldy from the left over fermenting juice.
- Most of all, 3-5 times a week. Simple activities like jogging or walking will help a lot in making you lose weight and be healthy.

Chapter 7 – Personal Tips

As mentioned in the introduction I wrote this book to share my personal experiences of how juicing has helped me with my help and become a regular part of my routine. I thought sharing how I do my routine would motivate you in seeing how easy juicing becomes once you make it a regular habit in your daily life.

A typical "work" day in my life:

Morning:

- Wake up between 6:30-7:00am
- Drink my "sour drink" a recipe for helping with my heart (sounds like a good book!!)
- Drink ½ glass of water while I prepare breakfast
- Breakfast = Oatmeal or some form of Oat Cereal most days with Strawberries, blueberries, raspberries, blackberries or a mix depending on what is the freshest available. Non-fat milk if I have cereal, just to make it easy to eat
- Vitamins – which I take with my morning "Red Detox Juice"
- Drink the other ½ glass of Water
- At the office I usually have a Ginseng Coffee
- Fill up my 16 ounce thermos with water to drink through the morning

Afternoon:

- ~12 noon - Lunch – Salad, healthy sandwich of turkey, lettuce, & tomato with mustard on healthy bread or roll
- On my way back from Lunch ~3 times a week I stop at the Juice place to get a mix of wheatgrass, vegetables, and fruit. There are a few other choices I sometimes get, but afternoon is a good time to have a wheatgrass juice
- I bring the juice up to the office and drink it through the afternoon
- I fill up the cup of juice with water after I finish the juice to drink more water with juicing flavor

Dinner:

- Get home and have ½ to 1 glass of water
- ~7pm – I usually have a low or non-carb dinner
- Dinner = pea soup, pumpkin soup, quinoa and salmon, tuna with celery & cashew nuts
- After dinner I take my herbal mix (another book I guess) followed by a glass of water
- If I am peck-ish (hungry) I have some fruit – grapes, a pear, a nectarine, or a peach
- I bring a full glass of water to sit next to the bed to drink while I read and in case I am thirst during the night

A weekend day in my life:

Morning:

- Wake up between 8:00-8:30am
- Drink my "sour drink" a recipe for helping with my heart
- Drink ½ glass of water while I prepare breakfast
- Breakfast = Oatmeal or some form of Oat Cereal most days with Strawberries, blueberries, raspberries, blackberries or a mix depending on what is the freshest available. Non-fat milk if I have cereal, just to make it easy to eat
- Vitamins – which I take with my morning "Red Detox Juice"
- Drink the other ½ glass of Water
- At the office I usually have a Ginseng Coffee
- Fill up my a glass with water to sit next to me while I work on my writing

Afternoon:

- ~12 noon - Lunch – I indulge and have some good home cooking, often Mediterranean diet food or Thai food
- Sometimes after Lunch make juice or stop by a juice place if I am out to get a second juice in and I try make it more a vegetable juice.
- I fill up the cup of juice with water after I finish the juice to drink more water with juicing flavor

Dinner:

- ~6pm – I have either a low-carb dinner or indulge a bit more (usually on Friday night or Saturday, but usually not both nights)

- Dinner = Most times like lunch Mediterranean food or Thai food
- After dinner I take my herbal mix followed by a glass of water
- If I am peck-ish (hungry) I have some fruit – grapes, a pear, a nectarine, or a peach
- I bring a full glass of water to sit next to the bed to drink while I read and in case I am thirst during the night

As you can see from my "typical routine" I have made juicing a regular part of every day. Even when I travel I try to get fresh juice in the hotel or find it during the day.

The fact is when I started juicing I was juicing 3-4 times a day for ~4 weeks straight and it made a big difference in my health. Then I added healthy Mediterranean food along with juicing into my routine. I feel my health was saved by juicing and I remember how feverish I was and how fatigued I felt with I had "mono". Others who have had "mono" had similar experiences, but use caffeine to this day to help them get through a typical day, I guess because they needed the boost to get through the afternoon fatigue that one with "mono" can experience. I started juicing due to a friend's advice and it gave me the energy I needed, so I did not want to use caffeine to help me with the extreme fatigue I was experiencing.

Now my routine is pretty easy and not complicated, yet I juice regularly and I love the energy juicing gives me. I rarely get a "common cold" or the flu compared to others around me, which I also contribute to juicing. I hope you are able to make juicing part of your life style as well!!

Conclusion

I hope you have garnered some helpful information about juicing and its benefits for the body. While there are many diets and other healthy eating habits introduced in the market, juicing has its own unique way of helping you live a healthy lifestyle. I for one am a great advocate of the juicing revolution and I hope that this will open the door for you to follow through and dedicate yourself to live a healthy lifestyle. Everything takes time, but you can make it part of your daily and weekly routine. Nothing can be done overnight that is why you have to have the motivation and determination to change. Although the saying health is wealth is a cliché, I have learned there are no riches in this world that could replace a healthy mind and body.

Be sure to make juicing a healthy habit for you and share with your whole family. Remember that it is better for your kids to start at an early age to develop the right habits. Consuming healthy foods coupled with exercise and a positive outlook in life is the best formula to live longer and happier. Enjoy preparing and coming up with your own concoctions. Be creative, be bold with flavors, and have fun doing it!

As a final word, remember: "A healthy outside starts from the inside." – Robert Urich

Good luck! Always be happy, always be healthy! Start TODAY!

Check Out Other Books

1) Take Charge of Your Health – Live to be 100 by Healing Yourself Naturally – by **Tammy Moore**

2) Rebuild Your Health with a Mediterranean Diet – Heart Healthy Eating Tips – by **Tammy Moore**